Anti inflammatory diet cookbook on a budget

Regain confidence and lose weight fast saving money with amazing and flavourful recipes, from beginners to advanced.

Joseph Monroe

Text Copyright © [Joseph Monroe]
All rights reserved. No part of this guide may be reproduced in any form without permission in writing from the publisher except in the case of brief quotations embodied in critical articles or reviews.

Legal & Disclaimer

The information contained in this book and its contents is not designed to replace or take the place of any form of medical or professional advice; and is not meant to replace the need for independent medical, financial, legal or other professional advice or services, as may be required. The content and information in this book have been provided for educational and entertainment purposes only.
The content and information contained in this book have been compiled from sources deemed reliable, and it is accurate to the best of the Author's knowledge, information, and belief. However, the author cannot guarantee its accuracy and validity and cannot be held liable for any errors and/or omissions. Further, changes are periodically made to this book as and when needed. Where appropriate and/or necessary, you must consult a professional (including but not limited to your doctor, attorney, financial advisor or such other professional advisor) before using any of the suggested remedies, techniques, or information in this book.
Upon using the contents and information contained in this book, you agree to hold harmless the Author from and against any damages, costs, and expenses, including any legal fees potentially resulting from the application of any of the information provided by this

book. This disclaimer applies to any loss, damages or injury caused by the use and application, whether directly or indirectly, of any advice or information presented, whether for breach of contract, tort, negligence, personal injury, criminal intent, or under any other cause of action.

You agree to accept all risks of using the information presented inside this book.

You agree that by continuing to read this book, where appropriate and/or necessary, you shall consult a professional (including but not limited to your doctor, attorney, or financial advisor or such other advisor as needed) before using any of the suggested remedies, techniques, or information in this book.

TABLE OF CONTENTS

TABLE OF CONTENTS   4

BREAKFAST   8

1. Perfect Barley Porridge   8
2. Morning Scrambled Turkey Eggs   10
3. Lovely Pumpkin Oats   12
4. Zucchini and Carrot Combo   14
5. Herb and Avocado Omelet   16
6. Tomato Egg Scramble   18
7. Choco-Nana Pancakes   20
8. Awesome Breakfast Parfait   22
9. Healthy Zucchini Stir Fry   24
10. Turmeric Protein Donuts   26

LUNCH 28

11. Greek Turkey Burgers with Tzatziki 28

12. Seared Ahi Tuna Poke Salad 30

13. One-Pan Eggs with Asparagus and Tomatoes 34

14. Anti-Inflammatory Buddha Bowl 36

15. Honey Ginger Shrimp Bowls 38

16. Salmon Cakes 41

17. Tuna Salad with White Beans 44

18. Chickpea Stuffed Butternut Squash 46

19. Clean Eating Egg Salad 49

20. White Bean Chili 51

DINNER 53

21. Shrimp and Vegetable Curry 53

22. Banana and Peanut Butter Detox 55

23. Escarole, Pineapple, and Apple Smoothie 56

24. Green and Leafy Ginger-Apple Drink	57
25. Nutty Pina Colada	58
26. Chai Tea Drink	59
27. Lemon-Mint Green Tea	60
28. Spicy Chicken Vegetable Soup	61
29. Lemon and Garlic Scallops	63
30. Walnut Encrusted Salmon	65

MEAT 67

31. Pork with Pineapple and Mango	67
32. Pork with Celery and Sprouts	69
33. Smoked Beef Sausage Bake with Broccoli	71
34. Keto Tacos with Bacon Sauce	73
35. Allspice Pork Mix	75
36. Pork with Parsley Mushrooms	77
37. Cinnamon Pork Mix	79

38. Balsamic Pork and Peaches	81
39. Pork with Scallions and Cauliflower	82
40. Pork with Spring Onions and Grapes	83
SOUP	**84**
41. Bacon & Cheese Soup	84
42. Beef and Veggie Soup	86
43. Broccoli Cheddar & Bacon Soup	88
44. Broccoli Soup with Gorgonzola Cheese	90
45. Brown Rice and Shitake Miso Soup with Scallion	92
46. Buffalo Sauce and Turkey Soup	94
47. Butternut Squash Soup with Shrimp	96
48. Cannellini Bean Soup	98
49. Carrot Broccoli Stew	100
50. Carrot, Ginger & Turmeric Soup	101

BREAKFAST

1. Perfect Barley Porridge

Preparation Time: 5 minutes

Cooking Time: 25 minutes

Serving: 4

Ingredients

- 1 cup barley
- 1 cup of wheat berries
- 2 cups unsweetened almond milk
- 2 cups of water
- Toppings, such as hazelnuts, honey, berry, etc.

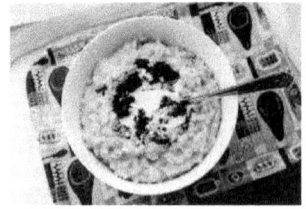

Directions:

1. Take a medium saucepan and place it over medium-high heat.
2. Place barley, almond milk, wheat berries, water and bring to a boil.

3. Reduce the heat to low and simmer for 25 minutes.
4. Divide amongst serving bowls and top with your desired toppings.
5. Serve and enjoy!

Nutrition: Calories: 295 Fat: 8g Carbohydrates: 56g Protein: 6g

2. Morning Scrambled Turkey Eggs

Preparation Time: 15 minutes

Cooking Time: 15 minutes

Serving: 2

Ingredients

- 1 tablespoon coconut oil
- 1 medium red bell pepper, diced
- ½ medium yellow onion, diced
- ¼ teaspoon hot pepper sauce
- 3 large free-range eggs
- ¼ teaspoon black pepper, freshly ground
- ¼ teaspoon salt

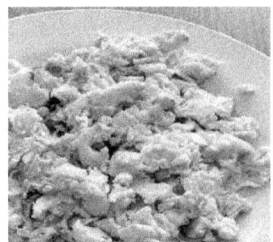

Directions:

1. Set a pan to medium-high heat and add coconut oil; let it heat up.
2. Add onions and sauté.
3. Add turkey and red pepper.

4. Cook until turkey is cooked.
5. Take a bowl and beat eggs, stir in salt and pepper.
6. Pour eggs in the pan with turkey and gently cook and scramble eggs.
7. Top with hot sauce and enjoy!

Nutrition: Calories: 435 Fat: 30g Carbohydrates: 34g Protein: 16g

3. Lovely Pumpkin Oats

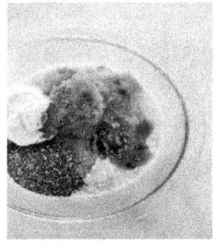

Preparation Time: 5 minutes

Cooking Time: 8 minutes

Serving: 3

Ingredients

- 1 cup quick-cooking rolled oats
- ¾ cup almond milk
- ½ cup canned pumpkin puree
- ¼ teaspoon pumpkin pie spice
- 1 teaspoon ground cinnamon

Directions:

1. Take a safe microwave bowl and add oats, almond milk, and microwave on high for 1-2 minutes.
2. Add more almond milk if needed to achieve your desired consistency.
3. Cook for 30 seconds more.

4. Stir in pumpkin puree, pumpkin pie spice, ground cinnamon.
5. Heat gently and enjoy!

Nutrition (Per Serving) Calories: 229 Fat: 4g Carbohydrates: 38g Protein: 10g

4. Zucchini and Carrot Combo

Preparation Time: 10 minutes

Cooking Time: 8 hours

Serving: 3

Ingredients

- ½ cup steel cut oats
- 1 cup of coconut milk
- 1 carrot, grated
- ¼ zucchini, grated
- Pinch of nutmeg
- ½ teaspoon cinnamon powder
- 2 tablespoons brown sugar
- ¼ cup pecans, chopped

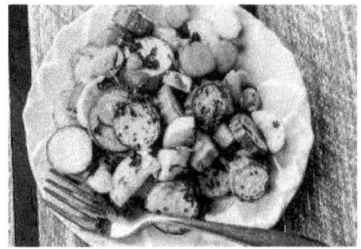

Directions:

1. Grease the Slow Cooker well.
2. Add oats, zucchini, milk, carrot, nutmeg, cloves, sugar, cinnamon, and stir well.

3. Place lid and cook on LOW for 8 hours.
4. Divide amongst serving bowls and enjoy!

Nutrition: Calories: 200 Fat: 4g Carbohydrates: 11g Protein: 5g

5. Herb and Avocado Omelet

Preparation Time: 2 minutes

Cooking Time: 10 minutes

Serving: 2

Ingredients

- 3 large free-range eggs
- ½ medium avocado, sliced
- ½ cup almonds, sliced
- Salt and pepper as needed

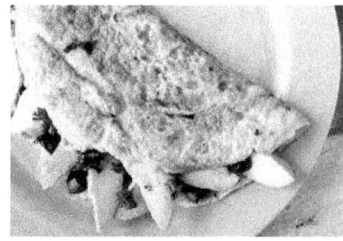

Directions:
1. Take a non-stick skillet and place it over medium-high heat.
2. Take a bowl and add eggs, beat the eggs.
3. Pour into the skillet and cook for 1 minute.
4. Lower heat to low and cook for 4 minutes.
5. Top the omelet with almonds and avocado.
6. Sprinkle salt and pepper and serve.
7. Enjoy!

Nutrition: Calories: 193 Fat: 15g Carbohydrates: 5g Protein: 10g

6. Tomato Egg Scramble

Preparation Time: 10 minutes

Cooking Time: 5 minutes

Serving: 2

Ingredients

- 2 whole eggs
- ½ cup fresh basil, chopped
- 2 tablespoons olive oil
- ½ teaspoon red pepper flakes, crushed
- 1 cup grape tomatoes, chopped
- Salt and pepper to taste

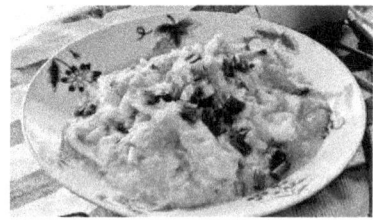

Directions:

1. Take a bowl and whisk in eggs, salt, pepper, red pepper flakes and mix well.
2. Add tomatoes, basil, and mix.
3. Take a skillet and place it over medium-high heat.
4. Add egg mixture and cook for 5 minutes and cooked and scrambled.

5. Enjoy!

Nutrition: Calories: 130 Fat: 10g Carbohydrates: 8g Protein: 1.8g

7. Choco-Nana Pancakes

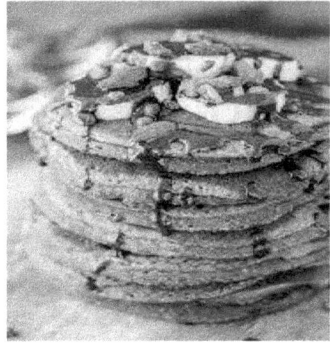

Preparation Time: 5 minutes

Cooking Time: 6 minutes

Serving: 2

Ingredients

- 2 large eggs, pasture-raised
- 2 large bananas, peeled and mashed
- 1 teaspoon pure vanilla extract
- 2 tablespoons almond butter
- 3 tablespoons cacao powder
- 1/8 teaspoon salt
- Coconut oil, for greasing

Directions:

1. Take a skillet and preheat on medium-low heat.
2. Grease the pan with coconut oil.

3. Add all ingredients to a food processor and blend until smooth.
4. Pour the batter into a skillet and make the pancake.
5. Cook for 3 minutes on each side. Serve and enjoy!

Nutrition: Calories: 303 Fat: 17g Carbohydrates: 36g Protein: 5g

8. Awesome Breakfast Parfait

Preparation Time: 5 minutes

Cooking Time: 0 minutes

Serving: 2

Ingredients

- 1 teaspoon sunflower seeds
- ½ cup low-fat milk
- 1 cup all-purpose flour
- 1 teaspoon vanilla
- 3 eggs, beaten
- 1 teaspoon baking soda
- 2 cups non-fat Greek yogurt

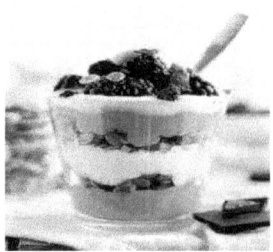

Directions:

1. Break up pretzels into small-sized portions and slice up the strawberries.
2. Add yogurt to the bottom of the glass and top with pretzels pieces and strawberries.

3. Add more yogurts and keep repeating until you have used up all ingredients.
4. Enjoy!

Nutrition: Calorie: 304 Fat: 1g Carbohydrates: 58g Protein: 15g

9. Healthy Zucchini Stir Fry

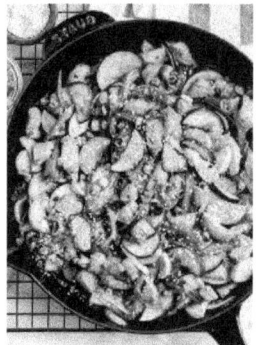

Preparation Time: 10 minutes

Cooking Time: 10 minutes

Serving: 4

Ingredients

- 2 tablespoons of heaping olive oil
- 1 whole medium-sized onion, sliced thinly
- 2 whole medium-sized zucchini, cut up into thin sized strips
- 2 heaping tablespoons of flavored teriyaki sauce, low sodium
- 1 whole tablespoon of coconut aminos
- 1 whole tablespoon of a sesame seed, toasted
- Ground pepper (black) as much as needed

Directions:

1. Take a skillet and place it over medium level heat.

2. Add onions and stir cook for 5 minutes.
3. Add your zucchini and stir cook for 1 minute more.
4. Gently add the sauces alongside the sesame seeds.
5. Cook for 5 minutes more until the zucchini are soft.
6. Finally, add in pepper and enjoy!

Nutrition: Calories: 110 Fat: 9g Carbohydrates: 8g Protein: 3g

10. Turmeric Protein Donuts

Preparation Time: 50 minutes
Cooking Time: 0 minutes
Serving: 8

Ingredients

- 1 ½ cups cashews, raw
- 2 tablespoons maple syrup
- ¼ teaspoon vanilla extract
- 1 tablespoon vanilla protein powder
- ½ cup Medjool dates pitted
- ¼ cup dark chocolate
- ½ cup coconut, shredded
- 1 teaspoon turmeric powder

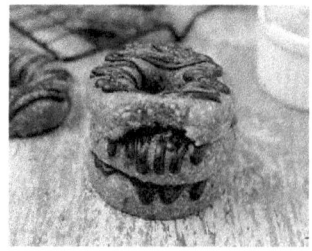

Directions:
1. Add all ingredients except chocolate to a food processor.
2. Pulse until smooth.

3. Roll batter 8 balls and press into silicone mold.
4. Place into the refrigerator for 30 minutes.
5. Make the chocolate topping.
6. Once done, remove the donuts from the mold.
7. Then drizzle with chocolate.
8. Serve and enjoy!

Nutrition: Calories: 320 Fat: 26g Carbohydrates: 20g Protein: 11g

LUNCH

11. Greek Turkey Burgers with Tzatziki

Preparation Time: 20 minutes
Cooking time 35 minutes
Servings: 4

Ingredients

- Turkey Burgers
- 1 tablespoon extra-virgin olive oil
- ½ cup sweet onion, minced
- 2 cloves garlic, minced
- 1 egg
- ½ cup chopped fresh parsley
- ½ teaspoon dried oregano
- ¼ teaspoon red pepper flakes
- 1 pound ground turkey
- ¾ cup bread crumbs
- Salt and freshly ground black pepper to taste
- 1 batch tzatziki sauce, for serving
- 4 hamburger buns, for serving

Directions
1. Preheat the oven to 375°F.
2. In a small skillet over medium, heat the oil and sauté the onions and garlic until soft. Set aside until they are cool.
3. Once cooled, mix the aromatics together with the egg, parsley, oregano, red pepper flakes, and ground turkey. Stir in the breadcrumbs, season with salt and pepper, and mix gently until completely combined. Form the mixture into four patties.
4. Spray an ovenproof skillet with non-stick cooking spray, then heat it over medium-high heat. Place the patties in the skillet and sear them on both sides, about 2 minutes on each side.
5. Move the skillet to the oven and cook for about 15 minutes, or until the burgers are cooked through.
6. While waiting for the burgers to cook, prepare the tzatziki sauce by mixing together all the ingredients.
7. When burgers are done, top with tzatziki sauce and whatever other toppings you desire.

Nutrition: Calories 326, fat 14 g, carbs 22 g, protein 27 g, sodium 109

12. Seared Ahi Tuna Poke Salad

Preparation Time: 20 minutes

Cooking time 105 minutes

Servings: 6

Ingredients

- Seared Ahi Tuna Poke
- 20 square wonton wrappers cut into strips (use corn tortillas to make this gluten free)
- 2 tablespoons olive oil
- ¼ cup soy sauce
- 1 teaspoon cornstarch
- ¼ cup pineapple juice
- ¼ cup honey
- 1 teaspoon chili garlic sauce or sriracha
- 2 tablespoons toasted sesame oil
- 6 (4 ounce) ahi tuna steaks
- 2 tablespoons black and white sesame seeds, toasted

For the salad

- 4–8 cups spring greens
- ½ cup fresh cilantro
- 1 cup fresh pineapple, diced

- 1 avocado, sliced
- 1 jalapeño or red chili, sliced
- Hula Ginger Vinaigrette
- (makes 1 ½ cups)
- ½ cup hot chili sesame oil or toasted sesame oil
- ¼ cup soy sauce
- 2 tablespoons pineapple juice
- 2 tablespoons rice vinegar
- 1 teaspoon chili garlic sauce or sriracha or more to taste
- 1 tablespoon tahini
- 1 lime, zested and juiced
- 2 teaspoons fresh ginger, grated
- 1 clove garlic, minced
- 1 tablespoon black and white sesame seeds, toasted

Directions

1. Preheat the oven to 400°F.
2. Grease a baking sheet with the olive oil and lay the wonton strips on it in a single layer. Sprinkle them with salt. Bake the strips for about 5 minutes, or until they

are golden brown and crispy. Set the finished strips to the side for now.

3. Pour the soy sauce into a small saucepan, then whisk in the cornstarch until incorporated. Stir in the pineapple juice, honey, and chili sauce.

4. Over medium-high heat, bring the mixture to a boil, then reduce the temperature and simmer for 3–5 minutes, or until the sauce begins to thicken. Set the thickened sauce aside.

5. Pour the sesame oil in a large skillet, and heat over high heat. Sear the tuna steaks for 1–2 minutes on each side. Brush the thickened soy sauce mixture over each side and cook another 1–2 minutes. Baste with sauce so each side is well covered. When the steaks are done, sprinkle each side with sesame seeds.

6. Prepare the salad. In a salad bowl, combine the greens, cilantro, pineapple, avocado, and jalapeño pepper. Toss to combine.

7. Make the vinaigrette by combining all the ingredients and whisking well.

8. Plate the greens, top with seared tuna and wonton crisps. Top with some of the vinaigrette, and serve.

Nutrition: (before adding vinaigrette)

Calories 447, fat 18 g, carbs 45 g, protein 32 g, sodium 856 mg

Nutrition: (serving = 2 tablespoons) (vinaigrette only)

Calories 103, fat 10 g, carbs 3 g, protein 1 g, sodium 346 mg

13. One-Pan Eggs with Asparagus and Tomatoes

Preparation Time: 10 minutes

Cooking time 20 minutes

Servings: 4

Ingredients:

- 2 pounds asparagus
- 1 pint cherry tomatoes
- 2 tablespoons olive oil
- 4 eggs
- 2 teaspoons chopped fresh thyme
- Salt and pepper to taste

Directions

1. Preheat the oven to 400°F.
2. Prepare a baking sheet by spraying it with non-stick cooking spray or olive oil.
3. Arrange the asparagus in an even layer on the sheet, and top it with the cherry tomatoes.
4. Pour the olive oil over the vegetables, and season them with salt and pepper.

5. Roast the vegetables until the asparagus is tender and tomatoes have softened (about 10 minutes).
6. Next, crack the eggs over the cooked vegetables and season with salt and pepper, and thyme.
7. Return the baking tray to the oven and cook until the egg whites are set, but the yolks are still soft.
8. Remove from oven and serve.

Nutrition: Calories 158, fat 11 g, carbs 13 g, protein 11 g

14. Anti-Inflammatory Buddha Bowl

Preparation Time: 10 minutes

Cooking time 30 minutes

Servings: 4

Ingredients

- 2 pounds cauliflower florets, stems removed
- 1 tablespoon plus one teaspoon extra-virgin olive oil, divided
- 1 teaspoon turmeric
- Salt and pepper
- 10 ounces kale, chopped
- 1 clove garlic, minced
- 8 medium beets, cooked, peeled, and chopped
- 2 avocados, cubed
- 2 cups fresh blueberries
- 1/3 cup raw walnuts, chopped

Directions

1. Preheat the oven to 425°F.
2. Cover a baking tray with foil and spray the foil with either coconut or olive oil.

3. Toss the cut cauliflower with 1 tablespoon of the olive oil and turmeric. Arrange it on the prepared baking tray. Season with salt and pepper and transfer the tray to the oven. Bake for about 30 minutes.
4. When the cauliflower is almost done, heat 1 teaspoon of olive oil in a large skillet. Add the kale and cook until it starts to wilt, then add the garlic.
5. When the cauliflower and kale are done, assemble the bowls. Start with kale, then top with cauliflower, beets, avocado, blueberries, and walnuts.
6. Serve, and enjoy!

Nutrition: Calories 450, fat 27 g, carbs 49 g, protein 13 g, sodium 377 mg

15. Honey Ginger Shrimp Bowls

Preparation Time: 20 minutes
Cooking time 6 minutes
Servings: 2

Ingredients

For the shrimp:

- 2 tablespoons honey
- 2 tablespoons coconut aminos or soy sauce
- 1 teaspoon fresh ginger, minced
- 2 cloves garlic, minced
- 12 ounces large uncooked shrimp, peeled and deveined
- 2 teaspoons avocado oil
- Lime, sea salt, and freshly ground pepper to taste

For the salad:

- 4 cups greens of your choice
- ½ cup shredded carrots
- ½ cup shredded radishes
- 4 green onions, sliced
- ¼ cup cilantro, chopped
- 1 avocado, sliced

For the dressing:

- 2 tablespoons lime juice
- 2 tablespoons extra-virgin olive oil
- 2 teaspoons coconut aminos
- 1 tablespoon honey
- 1 clove garlic, minced
- ½ teaspoon ginger powder
- Sea salt and pepper to taste

Directions

1. In a mixing bowl, whisk together the honey, coconut aminos (or soy sauce), ginger, and garlic as listed under shrimp ingredients.
2. Put the shrimp in a resealable bag and pour the marinade mixture in. Manipulate the bag to make sure all the shrimp are covered. Refrigerate while you are preparing the salad and dressing.
3. In a large skillet, heat the avocado oil over medium-high heat. When hot, add the shrimp and the marinade and cook for about 3 minutes. Turn the shrimp and cook for another 3 minutes or until the shrimp is fully cooked and sauce has thickened a bit. Season with lime juice, salt, and pepper.

4. Prepare the salad in a large bowl by mixing together all the ingredients.
5. Divide the salad into 2 servings, and top each with half the shrimp.
6. Prepare the dressing by whisking together all the ingredients.
7. Top the salad with dressing, and serve.

Nutrition: Calories 516, fat 32 g, carbs 47 g, protein 12 g, sodium 636 mg

16. Salmon Cakes

Preparation Time: 30 minutes

Cooking time 50 minutes

Servings: 5

Ingredients

- ½ pound fresh salmon
- 1 tablespoon olive oil
- Kosher salt and freshly ground black pepper
- ¼ cup olive oil
- ¼ cup unsalted butter
- 1 red onion, diced small
- 3 stalks celery, diced small
- 1 small red bell pepper, diced small
- 1 small yellow bell pepper, diced small
- ¼ cup minced fresh flat-leaf parsley
- 1 tablespoon capers, drained
- ½ teaspoon hot sauce
- ½ teaspoon Worcestershire sauce
- 1 teaspoon Old Bay seasoning
- 3 slices stale bread, crusts removed
- ½ cup mayonnaise

- 1 teaspoon mustard
- 2 eggs, lightly beaten

Directions

1. Preheat the oven to 375°F.
2. Cover a baking tray with parchment paper and place the salmon skin side down on the paper. Brush it with olive oil and bake for 15–20 minutes, or until it is just done.
3. Cool for 10 minutes, then put it in the fridge until it has cooled completely.
4. In a large skillet over medium-high, heat half the olive oil and half the butter. Add the onion, celery, peppers, parsley, capers, hot sauce, Worcestershire, Old Bay, and salt and pepper to taste. Let it cook about 15 minutes, or until the vegetables are soft. Remove it from the heat and let it cool.
5. Lightly toast the bread and crumble it up.
6. Using a fork, gently shred the cold salmon in a mixing bowl. Add the mayonnaise, mustard, and eggs. Then mix in the bread crumbs and the cooled vegetables.
7. Refrigerate the mixture for about 20 minutes, then shape it into patties. (It should make about 10 patties.)

8. In a large skillet, heat the remaining oil and butter. When it is hot, add the patties and cook for approximately 3–4 minutes on each side, until they are a nice golden brown. Transfer cooked patties to a paper towel lined plate to drain.

Nutrition: Calories 503, fat 43 g, carbs 12 g, protein 17 g, sodium 458 mg

17. Tuna Salad with White Beans

Preparation Time: 5 minutes
Cooking Time: 0 minutes
Servings: 2

Ingredients

- 1 can white tuna, packed in olive oil
- 1 (15 ounce) can white kidney or cannellini beans, rinsed and drained
- ½ cup red or sweet onion, minced
- ¼ cup fresh parsley, minced
- ¼ cup celery, minced
- 1 tablespoon fresh basil, minced
- 1 tablespoon extra-virgin olive oil
- 2 teaspoons apple cider vinegar
- Salt and pepper to taste

Directions

1. In a mixing bowl, break up the tuna in its oil. Add the beans.
2. Stir in the onion, parsley, basil, and celery. Mix everything together, ensuring that the tuna is well distributed.

3. Add the olive oil, vinegar, and salt and pepper. Stir again to combine.

Nutrition: Calories 276, fat 11 g, carbs 23 g, protein 26 g, sodium 526 mg

18. Chickpea Stuffed Butternut Squash

Preparation Time: 10 minutes

Cooking time 1 hour 15 minutes

Servings: 4

Ingredients

For the squash:

- 2 small butternut squashes, cut in half lengthwise and seeds removed
- 2 ½ tablespoons olive oil
- 1 ¼ cups fresh corn kernels

For the filling:

- 1 cup quinoa, cooked in 2 cups water or vegetable broth
- 1 (14 ounce) can chickpeas, drained
- ¼ cup red onion, diced
- 1 cup roasted red peppers, diced
- ½ cup fresh parsley, chopped
- ¾ cup pine nuts
- 1/3 cup olive oil
- ¼ cup apple cider vinegar
- Salt and freshly ground black pepper

- ½ cup shredded Gruyère cheese

Directions

1. Preheat the oven to 400°F.
2. Line 2 baking trays with aluminum foil and spray with non-stick cooking spray.
3. Rub the squash halves with some olive oil, and season them with salt and pepper. Arrange the squash (cut side down) on one of the prepared trays. Bake until the squash just begins to get tender (about 20–25 minutes).
4. Spread the corn kernels on the other baking tray and drizzle them with the remaining olive oil. Bake for 8–10 minutes, or until the corn starts to brown.
5. Prepare the filling. Place the cooked quinoa in a mixing bowl and toss in the roasted corn, chickpeas, red onion, red peppers, parsley, and pine nuts.
6. In a smaller bowl, whisk together the olive oil and apple cider vinegar. Season with salt and pepper to taste, and add it to the corn and chickpea mixture. Stir so that everything is well covered with the dressing.
7. Fill each squash half with some of the filling, sprinkle with shredded cheese, and place it back in the oven to cook until the cheese melts.

Nutrition: Calories 201, fat 9 g, carbs 29 g, protein 3 g, sodium 110 mg

19. Clean Eating Egg Salad

Preparation Time: 10 minutes

Cooking Time: 0 Minutes

Servings: 2

Ingredients:

- 6 organic pasture-raised eggs, hard-boiled
- 1 avocado
- ¼ cup of Greek yogurt
- 2 tablespoons of olive oil mayonnaise
- 1 teaspoon of fresh dill
- Sea salt to taste
- Lettuce for serving

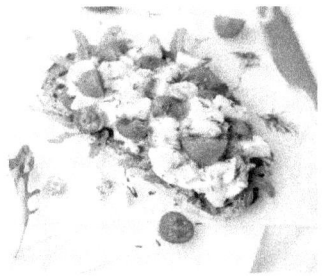

Directions:

1. Mash the hard-boiled eggs and avocado together.
2. Add in the Greek yogurt, olive oil mayonnaise, and fresh dill.
3. Season with sea salt. Serve on a bed of lettuce.

Nutrition: Total Carbohydrates 18g Dietary Fiber: 10g Protein: 23g Total Fat: 38g Calories: 486

20. White Bean Chili

Preparation Time: 10 minutes
Cooking Time: 20 Minutes
Servings: 4

Ingredients:

- ¼ cup extra-virgin olive oil
- 2 small onions, cut into ¼-inch dice
- 2 celery stalks, thinly sliced
- 2 small carrots, peeled and thinly sliced
- 2 garlic cloves, minced
- 2 teaspoons ground cumin
- 1½ teaspoons dried oregano
- 1 teaspoon salt
- ¼ teaspoon freshly ground black pepper
- 3 cups vegetable broth
- 1 (15½-ounce) can white beans, drained and rinsed
- ¼ finely chopped fresh flat-leaf parsley
- 2 teaspoons grated or minced lemon zest

Directions:
1. Heat-up the oil over high heat in a Dutch oven.

2. Add the onions, celery, carrots, and garlic and sauté until softened, 5 to 8 minutes.
3. Add the cumin, oregano, salt, and pepper and sauté to toast the spices, about 1 minute.
4. Put the broth and boil.
5. Simmer, add the beans, and cook, partially covered and occasionally stirring, for 5 minutes to develop the flavors.
6. Mix in the parsley and lemon zest and serve.

Nutrition: Calories 300 Total Fat: 15g Total Carbohydrates: 32g Sugar: 4g Fiber: 12g Protein: 12g Sodium: 1183mg

DINNER

21. Shrimp and Vegetable Curry

Preparation Time: 5 minutes

Cooking Time: 10 minutes

Servings: 4

Ingredients:

- 1 sliced onion
- 3 tablespoons of olive oil
- 2 teaspoons of curry powder
- 1 cup of coconut milk
- 1 cauliflower
- 1 lb. shrimp tails

Directions:

1. Add the onion to your oil.
2. Sauté to make it a bit soft.
3. Steam your vegetables in the meantime.
4. Add the curry seasoning, coconut milk, and spices if you want once the onion has become soft.
5. Cook for 2 minutes.
6. Include the shrimp. Cook for 5 minutes.

7. Serve with the steamed vegetables.

Nutrition Calories 491 Carbohydrates 11g Cholesterol 208mg Fat 39g Protein 24g Sugar 3g Fiber 5g Sodium 309mg

22. Banana and Peanut Butter Detox

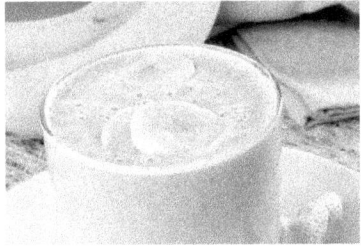

Preparation Time: 10 minutes

Cooking Time: 0 minute

Serving: 1

Ingredients

- 1/2 banana, frozen and fresh
- 2 tablespoons almond butter
- 1/4 cup dandelion green
- 1 cup beet greens
- 1/2 cup almond milk
- 6 ice cubes

Directions:

1. Add all ingredients in your blender
2. Blend it until you get a smooth and creamy mixture
3. Serve chilled and enjoy!

Nutrition: Calories: 366 Fat: 20g Carbohydrates: 44g Protein: 10g

23. Escarole, Pineapple, and Apple Smoothie

Preparation Time: 10 minutes

Cooking Time: 0 minute

Serving: 1

Ingredients

- 2 cups pineapple, cubed
- 2 apples, cored
- 8 ounces almond milk
- 1 head escarole lettuce
- 1 stalk celery

Directions:

1. Add all ingredients in your blender
2. Blend it until you get a smooth and creamy mixture
3. Serve chilled and enjoy!

Nutrition: Calories: 466 Fat: 8g Carbohydrates: 103g Protein: 8g

24. Green and Leafy Ginger-Apple Drink

Preparation Time: 10 minutes

Cooking Time: 0 minute

Serving: 1

Ingredients

- 1 medium apple, cored
- 2 medium carrots, chopped
- 2 large handfuls baby spinach
- 1 tablespoon ginger root, freshly grated
- 8 ounces of water, filtered

Directions:

1. Add all ingredients in your blender
2. Blend it until you get a smooth and creamy mixture
3. Serve chilled and enjoy!

Nutrition: Calories: 163 Fat: 0.1g Carbohydrates: 40g Protein: 3g

25. Nutty Pina Colada

Preparation Time: 10 minutes

Cooking Time: 0 minute

Serving: 1

Ingredients

- 1/2 banana
- 1/2 cup fresh pineapple, diced
- 1/4 teaspoon coconut extract
- 1/4 cup quick-cooking oats
- 5-6 ice cubes
- 1 container (6 ounces) Greek yogurt
- 1 cup almond milk
- 1 cup Swiss chard
- 1/4 cup Dandelion Greens

Directions:

1. Add all ingredients in your blender
2. Blend it until you get a smooth and creamy mixture
3. Serve chilled and enjoy!

Nutrition: Calories: 321 Fat: 6g Carbohydrates: 16g Protein: 15g

26. Chai Tea Drink

Preparation Time: 5 minutes

Cooking Time: 0 minute

Serving: 1

Ingredients:

- 1 cup almond milk
- 1 tablespoon honey
- 1 cup boiling water
- ¼ teaspoon cacao powder
- 1 green tea bag

Directions:

1. Take a large mug, add a tea bag and hot water
2. Leave it for 5 minutes
3. Discard tea bag and stir in cacao powder and honey
4. Mix them well
5. Stir in cold almond milk
6. Serve and enjoy!

Nutrition: Calories: 216 Fat: 8g Carbohydrates: 29g Protein: 8g

27. Lemon-Mint Green Tea

Preparation Time: 10 minutes

Cooking Time: 0 minute

Serving: 1

Ingredients

- 2 lemon slices
- 1 green tea bag
- 3 mint leaves
- 1 tablespoon honey
- 2 cups boiling water

Directions:

1. Take a large mug, add lemon slices, tea bag, and hot water
2. Leave it for 10 minutes
3. Discard tea bag and stir in lemon slices and honey
4. Mix them well
5. Stir in mint leaves
6. Serve and enjoy!

Nutrition: Calories: 87 Fat: 0.2g Carbohydrates: 24g Protein: 0.8g

28. Spicy Chicken Vegetable Soup

Preparation Time: 10 minutes

Cooking Time: 25 minutes

Serving: 4

Ingredients

- 1-pound chicken, skinless
- 1 teaspoon basil, dried
- 1 small onion, diced
- 1 can tomatoes, diced
- 2 cups vegetable, frozen
- 3 bay leaves
- 1 garlic clove, minced
- 1 and ½ cups sweet potatoes, cubed
- ½ teaspoon red chili pepper flakes
- 1 jar spicy tomato sauce
- ½ teaspoon of sea salt
- 2 cups chicken broth

Directions:

1. Add all ingredients in your Dutch oven, mix them well
2. Season with salt and pepper
3. Simmer for 15 minutes

4. Then cook 10 minutes
5. Serve warm and enjoy!

Nutrition: Calories: 279 Fat: 11g Carbohydrates: 18g Protein: 27g

29. Lemon and Garlic Scallops

Preparation Time: 10 minutes

Cooking Time: 5 minutes

Serving: 4

Ingredients

- 1 tablespoon olive oil
- 1 and ¼ pounds dried scallops
- 2 tablespoons all-purpose flour
- ¼ teaspoon sunflower seeds
- 4-5 garlic cloves, minced
- 1 scallion, chopped
- 1 pinch of ground sage
- 1 lemon juice
- 2 tablespoons parsley, chopped

Directions:

1. Take a non-stick skillet and place it over medium-high heat
2. Add oil and allow the oil to heat up
3. Take a medium-sized bowl and add scallops alongside sunflower seeds and flour

4. Place the scallops in the skillet and add scallions, garlic, and sage
5. Sauté for 3-4 minutes until they show an opaque texture
6. Stir in lemon juice and parsley
7. Remove heat and serve hot!

Nutrition: Calories: 151 Fat: 4g Carbohydrates: 10g Protein: 18g

30. Walnut Encrusted Salmon

Preparation Time: 10 minutes

Cooking Time: 14 minutes

Servings: 34

Ingredients

- ½ cup walnuts
- 2 tablespoons stevia
- ½ tablespoon Dijon mustard
- ¼ teaspoon dill
- 2 Salmon fillets (3 ounces each)
- 1 tablespoon olive oil
- Sunflower seeds and pepper to taste

Directions:

1. Preheat your oven to 350 degrees F
2. Add walnuts, mustard, stevia to a food processor and process until your desired consistency is achieved
3. Take a frying pan and place it over medium heat
4. Add oil and let it heat up
5. Add salmon and sear for 3 minutes
6. Add walnut mix and coat well

7. Transfer coated salmon to the baking sheet, bake in the oven for 8 minutes
8. Serve and enjoy!

Nutrition: Calories: 373 Fat: 43g Carbohydrates: 4g Protein: 20g

MEAT

31. Pork with Pineapple and Mango

Preparation Time: 10 minutes

Cooking Time: 40 minutes

Servings: 4

Ingredients:

- 4 pork chops
- 2 tablespoons olive oil
- ½ cup vegetable stock
- 4 scallions, chopped
- 1 cup pineapple, peeled and cubed
- 1 mango, peeled and cubed
- 4 tablespoons lime juice
- 1 handful basil, chopped
- A pinch of salt and cayenne pepper

Directions:

1. Heat up a pan with the oil over medium heat, add the scallions and the meat and brown for 5 minutes.

2. Add the pineapple and the other ingredients, toss, cook over medium heat for 35 minutes more, divide between plates and serve.

Nutrition: calories 250, fat 5, fiber 6, carbs 8, protein 17

32. Pork with Celery and Sprouts

Preparation Time: 10 minutes

Cooking Time: 40 minutes

Servings: 4

Ingredients:

- 2 pounds pork stew meat, roughly cubed
- 2 tablespoons olive oil
- 2 tablespoons lemon juice
- 5 garlic cloves, minced
- 2 stalks celery, chopped
- 1 cup Brussels sprouts, trimmed and halved
- A pinch of salt and black pepper
- ½ teaspoon cinnamon powder
- 2 tablespoons parsley, chopped

Directions:

1. Heat up a pan with the oil over medium-high heat, add the garlic and the meat and brown for 5 minutes.
2. Add the celery and the other ingredients, toss, introduce the pan in the oven and cook at 400 degrees F for 35 minutes more.
3. Divide the mix between plates and serve.

Nutrition: calories 284, fat 4, fiber 4, carbs 9, protein 15

33. Smoked Beef Sausage Bake with Broccoli

Preparation Time: 45 minutes

Cooking Time: 40 minutes

Servings: 4

Ingredients

- 1 red bell pepper, thinly sliced
- 2 shallots, chopped
- 1 cup broccoli, broken into florets
- 4 smoked beef sausages, sliced
- 1 green bell pepper, thinly sliced
- 2 tablespoons fresh parsley, roughly chopped
- 2 garlic cloves, minced
- 1/2 teaspoon ground bay leaf
- Salt and black pepper, to taste
- 1 teaspoon marjoram
- 6 eggs, whisked

Directions

1. Begin by preheating your oven to 3700F.
2. Heat up a nonstick skillet using a moderate flame; now, Heat the sausage for 3 minutes, stirring regularly.

3. Include the peppers, shallots, broccoli, and garlic; continue cooking for about 5 minutes. Season with marjoram, salt, pepper and ground bay leaf.
4. Move the sausage mixture to a previously greased baking dish. Pour the whisked eggs over it. Bake for 35 minutes. Enjoy garnished with fresh parsley.

Nutrition: Calories 289, Protein 19.8g ,Fat 19.7g ,Carbs 6.3g ,Sugar 2.4g

34. Keto Tacos with Bacon Sauce

Preparation Time: 30 minutes

Cooking Time: 40 minutes

Servings: 4

Ingredients

- 1 ½ cups ground beef
- 2 jalapeno peppers, minced
- 2 Campari tomatoes, crushed
- 1/2 teaspoon ground cumin
- 6 slices bacon, chopped
- 2 teaspoon champagne vinegar
- 1/2 teaspoon onion powder
- 1/2 teaspoon celery salt
- 1 ½ cups Cotija cheese, shredded
- Salt and ground black pepper, to taste
- 1/2 cup bone broth
- 3 tablespoons tomato paste

Directions

1. Begin by preheating your oven to 3900F. Spritz a baking pan with the aid of a nonstick cooking spray.

2. Spread 6 (six piles of Cotija cheese on the baking pan; bake for about 15 minutes; allow taco shells to cool down for some minutes.
3. In a nonstick skillet, brown the beef for the duration of about 4 to 5 minutes crumbling with a spatula. Include crushed pepper, tomatoes, salt, celery salt, onion powder, and ground cumin.
4. Heat until everything is cooked through.
5. Now, make the sauce by cooking the bacon for the duration of 2 to 3 minutes stirring continually. Include the remaining ingredients and heat until everything comes together.
6. After the above, assemble your tacos. Share the meat mixture among 6 taco shells; top with the bacon sauce. Bon appétit!

Nutrition: Calories 258, Protein 16.3g, Fat 19.3g, Carbs 5g, Sugar 2.9g

35. Allspice Pork Mix

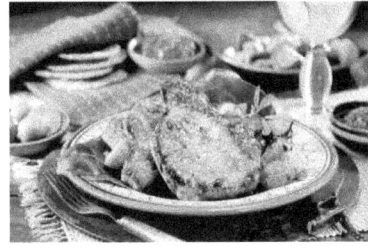

Preparation Time: 10 minutes

Cooking Time: 1 hour

Servings: 4

Ingredients:

- 2 tablespoons olive oil
- 2 pounds pork stew meat, cubed
- 1 teaspoon cumin, ground
- 1 tablespoon sage, chopped
- 1 yellow onion, chopped
- 1 cup vegetable stock
- A pinch of salt and black pepper
- 1 teaspoon chili pepper flakes, dried
- ½ teaspoon allspice, ground

Directions:

1. Heat up a pan with the oil over medium-high heat, add the onion and the meat and brown for 10 minutes.

2. Add the rest of the ingredients, toss, introduce in the oven and bake at 390 degrees F for 50 minutes.
3. Divide everything between plates and serve.

Nutrition: calories 261, fat 4, fiber 7, carbs 12, protein 18

36. Pork with Parsley Mushrooms

Preparation Time: 10 minutes

Cooking Time: 8 hours and 10 minutes

Servings: 4

Ingredients:

- 1 green bell pepper, chopped
- 1 red bell pepper, chopped
- 1 cup white mushrooms, sliced
- 1 pound pork stew meat, cubed
- 1 yellow onion, chopped
- 2 tablespoons olive oil
- Salt and black pepper to the taste
- 1 cup tomatoes, chopped
- 1 tablespoon parsley, chopped
- 2 teaspoons chili powder

Directions:

1. Heat up a pan with the oil over medium heat, add the onion and the mushrooms and sauté for 5 minutes.
2. Add the meat and brown for 5 minutes more.

3. Transfer everything to your slow cooker, add the rest of the ingredients, toss, put the lid on and cook on Low for 8 hours.
4. Divide everything between plates and serve.

Nutrition: calories 274, fat 6, fiber 3, carbs 11, protein 24

37. Cinnamon Pork Mix

Preparation Time: 10 minutes

Cooking Time: 1 hour

Servings: 4

Ingredients:

- 2 pounds pork stew meat, cubed
- 2 tablespoons olive oil
- 1 yellow onion, chopped
- 2 avocados, peeled, pitted and sliced
- 1 tablespoon chili powder
- Salt and black pepper to the taste
- 1 teaspoon cumin, ground
- ½ teaspoon cinnamon powder
- A pinch of cayenne pepper
- ½ cup vegetable stock
- ½ cup parsley, chopped

Directions:

1. Heat up a pan with the oil over medium-high heat, add the onion and the meat and brown for 10 minutes stirring often.

2. Add the avocados and the other ingredients toss, introduce the pan in the oven and bake at 390 degrees F for 50 minutes.
3. Divide the mix between plates and serve.

Nutrition: calories 300, fat 7, fiber 6, carbs 12, protein 18

38. Balsamic Pork and Peaches

Preparation Time: 10 minutes

Cooking Time: 45 minutes

Servings: 4

Ingredients:

- 2 peaches, cubed
- 1 cup red cabbage, shredded
- 2 pounds pork stew meat, cubed
- 2 tablespoons olive oil
- 4 scallions, chopped
- 1 tablespoon balsamic vinegar
- A pinch of salt and black pepper
- 1 tablespoon cilantro, chopped

Directions:

1. Heat up a pan with the oil over medium-high heat, add the scallions and the meat and brown for 10 minutes.
2. Add the peaches and the other ingredients, toss and cook over medium heat for 35 minutes.
3. Divide everything between plates and serve.

Nutrition: calories 260, fat 5, fiber 4, carbs 12, protein 14

39. Pork with Scallions and Cauliflower

Preparation Time: 10 minutes

Cooking Time: 8 hours

Servings: 4

Ingredients:

- 2 pounds pork roast, sliced
- 4 scallions, chopped
- 2 garlic cloves, minced
- 1 yellow onion, chopped
- 2 tablespoons olive oil
- 1 cup cauliflower florets
- ½ cup vegetable stock
- A pinch of salt and black pepper
- A pinch of red chili pepper flakes

Directions:

1. In your slow cooker, mix the pork roast with the scallions, the garlic and the other ingredients, toss, put the lid on and cook on Low for 8 hours.
2. Divide everything between plates and serve.

Nutrition: calories 556, fat 29, fiber 1.7, carbs 6, protein 65.8

40. Pork with Spring Onions and Grapes

Preparation Time: 10 minutes
Cooking Time: 40 minutes
Servings: 6

Ingredients:

- 2 pounds pork stew meat, cubed
- 2 spring onions, chopped
- 1 cup grapes, halved
- 2 tablespoons olive oil
- ¼ teaspoon coriander, ground
- ¼ teaspoon smoked paprika
- ¼ cup coconut aminos
- A pinch of salt and black pepper

Directions:

1. Heat up a pan with the oil over medium heat, add the onions and the meat and brown for 10 minutes.
2. Add the rest of the ingredients, toss, cook over medium heat for 30 minutes more, divide between plates and serve.

Nutrition: calories 574, fat 29, fiber 0.5, carbs 7.6, protein 66.7

SOUP

41. Bacon & Cheese Soup

Preparation Time: fifteen minutes

Cooking Time: forty minutes

Servings: 6

Ingredients:

- ½ cup sour cream, for serving
- ½ teaspoon cumin
- ½ teaspoon onion powder
- ½ teaspoon paprika
- 1 cup heavy cream
- 1 cup shredded cheddar cheese
- 1 pound of lean ground beef
- 1 tablespoon coconut oil, for cooking
- 1 teaspoon garlic powder
- 1 yellow onion, chopped
- 6 cups beef broth
- 6 slices uncured bacon

Directions:

1. Put in the coconut oil to a frying pan and cook the bacon until crunchy. Allow the bacon to cool and cut into little pieces. Set aside.
2. Once cooked, put in the lean ground beef to the same frying pan with the bacon fat and cook until browned.
3. Put in the onions and cook for an extra two to three minutes.
4. Put in all the ingredients minus the bacon, heavy cream, sour cream and cheese to a stockpot and stir. Cook for about twenty-five minutes.
5. Warm the heavy cream, and then put in the warmed cream and cheese and serve with the bacon and a spoonful of sour cream.

Nutrition: Calories: 498 , Carbohydrates: 5g , Fiber: 1g Net , Carbohydrates: 4g , Fat: 34g , Protein: 41g

42. Beef and Veggie Soup

Preparation Time: ten minutes
Cooking Time: twenty minutes
Servings: 8

Ingredients:

- ½ cup heavy whipping cream
- ½ cup onion, chopped
- 1 (8 ounces / 227 g) package cream cheese, softened
- 1 pound (454 g) ground beef
- 1 tablespoon ground cumin
- 1 teaspoon chili powder
- 2 (10 ounces / 284 g) cans diced tomatoes and green chiles
- 2 (14.5 ounces / 411 g) cans beef broth
- 2 cloves garlic, minced
- 2 teaspoons salt, or to taste

Directions:

1. Position the ground beef, chopped onion, and garlic in a pot, stir until blended well. Cook on moderate to high heat for five to seven minutes or until the beef is thoroughly browned. Stir continuously.

2. Discard the grease extract from the beef, then put in chili powder and cumin, and cook for an extra two minutes. Stir continuously.
3. Put in the cream cheese to the pot and cook for three to five minutes more, then fold in the tomatoes and green chiles, beef broth, heavy whipping cream, and salt, and cook for about ten minutes to cook through. Keep stirring during the cooking.
4. Serve the soup in a big serving container. Allow to stand for a couple of minutes before you serve.

Nutrition: calories: 288 , total fat: 24g , carbs: 5.4g , protein: 13.4g , Cholesterol: 85mg , Sodium: 1310mg

43. Broccoli Cheddar & Bacon Soup

Preparation Time: ten minutes

Cooking Time: ten minutes

Servings: 6

Ingredients:

- ¼ teaspoon black pepper
- ½ teaspoon salt
- ½ white onion, chopped
- 1 cup broccoli florets finely chopped
- 1 cup heavy cream
- 1 cup shredded cheddar cheese
- 2 cloves garlic, chopped
- 2 cups chicken broth
- 3 slices cooked bacon, crumbled for serving

Directions:

1. Put in all the ingredients minus the heavy cream, cheddar cheese and bacon to a stockpot on moderate heat.
2. Heat to a simmer and cook for 5 minutes.

3. Warm the cream, and then put in the warm cream and cheddar cheese. Whisk until the desired smoothness is achieved.
4. Serve with crumbled bacon.

Nutrition: Calories: 220 , Carbohydrates: 4g , Fiber: 1g Net , Carbohydrates: 3g , Fat: 18g , Protein: 11g

44. Broccoli Soup with Gorgonzola Cheese

Preparation Time: ten minutes
Cooking Time: thirty minutes
Servings: 4

Ingredients:

- ½ cup 18% cream
- 1 big broccoli, divided into little roses
- 1 flat teaspoon of sweet pepper
- 1 onion, diced
- 1 tablespoon of chopped fresh basil
- 1 tablespoon of chopped parsley
- 1 tablespoon of oil
- 150 g Gorgonzola cheese, diced
- 2 potatoes, peeled and diced
- 4 tablespoons of almond flakes roasted in a dry pan
- 5 garlic cloves, chopped
- 750 ml broth
- a pinch of sugar
- pumpkin oil (not necessary)
- salt and pepper

Directions:

1. In a big deep cooking pan, warm the oil on moderate heat, put the onion and garlic, and fry it until the vitrified glass onion.
2. Then put the broccoli with potatoes, pour the broth and cook for approximately fifteen-twenty minutes until the vegetables become tender. Put in basil, parsley, sugar, pepper, and pepper to taste.
3. Put in cheese and cream, and when the cheese dissolves, blend with a blender until the desired smoothness is achieved. Sprinkle with salt and pepper if required.
4. Serve the soup sprinkled with almond flakes and sprinkled with pumpkin oil.

Nutrition: Calories: 382 kcal , Protein: 13.06 g , Fat: 18.93 g , Carbohydrates: 41.65 g

45. Brown Rice and Shitake Miso Soup with Scallion

Preparation Time: ten minutes

Cooking Time: forty-five minutes

Servings: 4

Ingredients:

- ½ teaspoon salt
- 1 (1½-inch) piece fresh ginger, peeled and cut
- 1 cup medium-grain brown rice
- 1 cup thinly cut shiitake mushroom caps
- 1 garlic clove, minced
- 1 tablespoon white miso
- 2 scallions, thinly cut
- 2 tablespoons finely chopped fresh cilantro
- 2 tablespoons sesame oil

Directions:

1. In a large pot, heat the oil on moderate to high heat.
2. Put in the mushrooms, garlic, and ginger and sauté until the mushrooms start to tenderize, approximately five minutes.
3. Place the rice and stir to uniformly coat with the oil.

4. Put in 2 cups of water and salt and place it to its boiling point.
5. Reduce the heat then cook until the rice is soft, thirty to forty minutes.
6. Use a little of the soup broth to tenderize the miso, then mix it into the pot until well mixed.
7. Stir in the scallions and cilantro, then serve.

Nutrition: Calories: 265 , Total Fat: 8g , Total Carbohydrates: 43g , Sugar: 2g , Fiber: 3g , Protein: 5g , Sodium: 456mg

46. Buffalo Sauce and Turkey Soup

Preparation Time: five minutes

Cooking Time: ten minutes

Servings: Servings 4

Ingredients:

- 1/3 cup buffalo sauce
- 2 cups turkey, cooked, shredded
- 3 tablespoons butter, melted
- 4 cups chicken broth
- 4 ounces (113 g) cream cheese
- 4 tablespoons cilantro, chopped
- From The Cupboard:
- Salt and freshly ground black pepper, to taste

Directions:

1. Place the buffalo sauce, cream cheese, and melted butter in a blender, and process until the desired smoothness is achieved.
2. Pour the buffalo sauce mixture in a deep cooking pan, and put in the chicken broth. Heat the soup using high heat until hot and nearly boil off but not boil. Keep stirring during the heating.

3. Put in the shredded turkey, and drizzle with salt and black pepper. Cook for five minutes or until the desired smoothness is achieved. Stir continuously.
4. Ladle the soup into a big container and top with chopped cilantro before you serve.

Nutrition: calories: 409 , total fat: 29.7g , net carbs: 9.2g , protein: 26.4g

47. Butternut Squash Soup with Shrimp

Preparation Time: 10 minutes

Cooking Time: 20minutes

Servings: 4

Ingredients:

- ¼ cup slivered almonds (not necessary)
- ¼ teaspoon freshly ground black pepper
- 1 cup unsweetened almond milk
- 1 garlic clove, cut
- 1 pound cooked peeled shrimp, thawed if required
- 1 small red onion, finely chopped
- 1 teaspoon salt
- 1 teaspoon turmeric
- 2 cups peeled butternut squash cut into ¼-inch dice
- 2 tablespoons finely chopped fresh flat-leaf parsley
- 2 teaspoons grated or minced lemon zest
- 3 cups vegetable broth
- 3 tablespoons unsalted butter

Directions:

1. In a large pot, melt the butter on high heat.

2. Put in the onion, garlic, turmeric, salt, and pepper and sauté until the vegetables are tender and translucent, five to seven minutes.
3. Put in the broth and squash and bring to its boiling point.
4. Reduce the heat and cook until the squash has tenderized, approximately five minutes.
5. Put in the shrimp and almond milk and cook until thoroughly heated, approximately 2 minutes.
6. Drizzle with the almonds (if using), parsley, and lemon zest before you serve.

Nutrition: Calories: 275 , Total Fat: 12g , Total Carbohydrates: 12g , Sugar: 3g , Fiber: 2g; , Protein: 30g , Sodium: 1665mg

48. Cannellini Bean Soup

Preparation Time: twenty-five minutes
Cooking Time: thirty minutes
Servings: 6

Ingredients:

- 1 bunch red Swiss chard
- 1 cannellini beans
- 1 clove garlic (minced)
- 1 onion (chopped)
- 1 tablespoon extra-virgin olive oil
- 1/4 teaspoon nutmeg (grated)
- 1/8 teaspoon red pepper flakes (crushed)
- 2 ounces Parmesan cheese rind
- 2 slices smoked bacon (chopped)
- 2 tablespoons chopped sun-dried tomatoes
- 5 big sage leaves (minced)
- 5 leaves basil (chopped)
- 6 cups chicken broth

Directions:

1. Cook the bacon with garlic, onion, nutmeg, and red pepper flakes for five minutes.

2. Pour in beans, chicken broth, sun-dried tomatoes, and Parmesan cheese rind, simmering for about ten minutes.
3. Put in the cut chard and chard leaves into the soup.
4. Simmer and then put in into bowls with a sprinkle of oil and Parmesan cheese.

Nutrition: Calories: 215 kcal , Carbohydrates: 23 g , Fat: 10 g , Protein: 9.7 g

49. Carrot Broccoli Stew

Preparation Time: ten minutes

Cooking Time: forty-five minutes

Servings: 3

Ingredients:

- 1 cup Broccoli, florets
- 1 cup Carrots, cut
- 1 cup Heavy Cream
- 3 cups Chicken broth
- Salt and black pepper to taste

Directions:

1. Put in florets, cream, carrots, salt, and chicken broth; toss thoroughly. Secure the lid and cook on Meat/Stew mode for forty minutes on High. When ready, do a quick pressure release.
2. Move into serving bowls and drizzle black pepper on top.

Nutrition: Calories 145 , Protein: 1.5g , Carbs: 1.2g

50. Carrot, Ginger & Turmeric Soup

Preparation Time: fifteen minutes

Cooking Time: forty minutes

Servings: 8

Ingredients:

- ¼ cup full-fat unsweetened coconut milk
- ¾ pound carrots, peeled and chopped
- 1 sweet yellow onion, chopped
- 1 teaspoon ground turmeric
- 2 cloves garlic, chopped
- 2 teaspoons grated ginger
- 6 cups vegetable broth
- Pinch of sea salt & pepper, to taste

Directions:

1. Put in all the ingredients minus the coconut milk to a stockpot on moderate heat and bring to its boiling point. Reduce to a simmer and cook for forty minutes or until the carrots are soft.
2. Use an immersion blender and blend the soup until the desired smoothness is achieved. Mix in the coconut milk.

3. Enjoy immediately and freeze any remaining.

Nutrition: Calories: 73 , Carbohydrates: 7g , Fiber: 2g Net , Carbohydrates: 5g , Fat: 3g , Protein: 4g

CPSIA information can be obtained
at www.ICGtesting.com
Printed in the USA
LVHW051137110621
689903LV00006B/637